SOMATIC EXERCISES FOR WEIGHT LOSS 2024

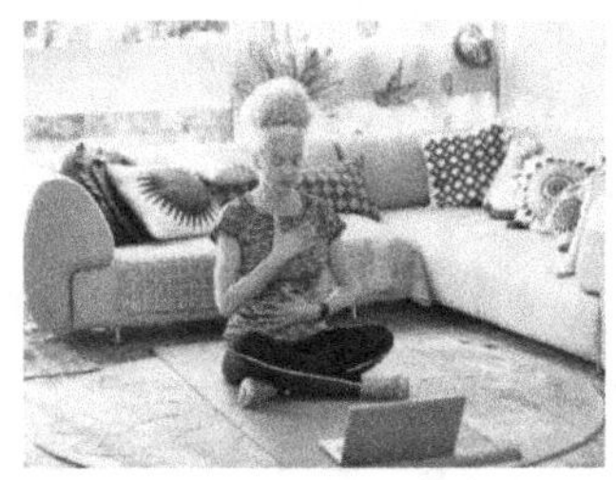

Complete Workout Plan to Release Stress and Anxiety for Your Body

ROBERT H WOODS

Table of Contents

4 Somatic Exercises For Weight Loss

Introduction

Starting a weight reduction journey is often fraught with difficulties and false beliefs. The pursuit of health involves more than just losing weight; it also involves adopting a way of life that balances the body and the mind. This is where the emphasis of this book, the somatic exercises, comes in.

Somatic exercises focus interior bodily sense and experience, offering a unique approach to fitness and well-being. The Greek word "soma," from which the term "somatic" is derived, refers to "the living body." Somatic exercises promote a deeper connection with one's body, promoting awareness and relieving tension, in contrast to typical workout programs that often focus exterior appearance and repetitive action.

Somatic activities are effective in helping us lose weight because they change the way we think about our body. These exercises assist to re-train the body to move more smoothly and effectively by concentrating on the sensory-motor system. This helps with weight control by enhancing metabolic processes and promoting better posture and flexibility.

We will examine the foundations of somatic movement and how they relate to weight reduction in this book. You'll study about Sensory Motor Amnesia, a disorder in which certain muscles grow so used to using themselves in a particular way that they lose the ability to use them in other ways. You may activate these muscles by somatic workouts, which will result in more energetic and dynamic motions.

We will lead you through a progression of somatic exercises, beginning with simple motions that everyone can do at home and working up to more complex methods. Every workout program is designed with the goals of enhancing muscle performance, fostering relaxation, and raising body awareness—all of which are crucial for reaching and maintaining a healthy weight.

Additionally, this book will explore how to include somatic workouts into your daily routine to help you achieve your weight reduction goals in a more sustainable and achievable way. We will also discuss mindful eating as a way to enhance your somatic practice and the significance of nutrition.

Turning the pages will reveal that somatic exercises are a route to deciphering your body's signals and language, not merely a set of actions. With this information at your disposal, you can make wise decisions about your health and wellbeing, which will help you live a more balanced and satisfying life.

Come along on this life-changing trip with us as we uncover the potential of somatic workouts to help you lose weight. Forget about the numbers on the scale; what matters is forging a healthy, long-lasting connection with your body.

Chapter 1: Comprehending Somatic Activities

A kind of movement therapy known as somatic exercises places more emphasis on the inner sensation of movement than on performance or outward look. This method is based on the idea of somatics, which is the study of the self from the viewpoint of one's actual experience in the body, including the relationship between the mind and body.

Regaining voluntary control over the body's musculature via movement and awareness is the fundamental principle of somatic exercises. These exercises aim to help people relieve chronic muscular tension, enhance proprioception (the awareness of one's own movement and posture), and re-educate their nervous system. This is accomplished by concentrating on the feelings that surface during movement as opposed to the volume or level of exertion.

Key components of somatic exercises include the following:

1. Sensory Awareness: Somatic practices promote an enhanced awareness of the body's feelings, including pain, tension, and relaxation. This awareness is essential for figuring out where in the body stress is being held without need and for learning how to release it.

2. Muscle relaxation: Somatic exercises help with the relaxation of taut muscles with mild, deliberate motions; this is often called "pandiculation." By progressively relaxing and tightening the muscles, this technique might assist to restore the muscle length and lessen discomfort.

3. Movement Re-education: Retraining the body to move more easily and effectively is the goal of many somatic exercises. Those who have acquired bad movement habits or sustained injuries that have changed their natural movement patterns can especially benefit from this.

4. Mind-Body Integration: Somatic exercises include mental aspects in addition to physical ones. Through focusing on the quality of movement and the emotions that accompany it, practitioners may strengthen the connection between their body and mind, resulting in increased overall harmony and wellbeing.

5. Self-Regulation: The capacity to control one's own nervous system is a major advantage of somatic exercises. Through deliberate muscle relaxation and stress reduction, people may affect their autonomic nervous system, which regulates involuntary body processes like digestion and heart rate.

6. Adaptability: Somatic exercises are very flexible and may be tailored to accommodate people of different skill levels and fitness levels. They are accessible to a broad audience since they may be done anywhere and don't need specialized equipment.

To sum up, somatic exercises are an effective means of reestablishing a connection with the body, letting go of stress, and enhancing mobility. They are an essential tool for anybody trying to improve their physical and mental health, and they are also a key component of a weight reduction strategy that is holistic. Your body may become more receptive and attuned by including somatic exercises in your routine, which will open the door to a healthier and more balanced existence.

How the Mind and Body Affect Weight Loss

1. The Mind-Body Link in Losing Weight:
    Many people think that losing weight is just a physical process that involves food and exercise. Nonetheless, reaching and maintaining a healthy weight greatly depends on the mind-body link. The complex relationship that exists between our emotional and mental states and our physical health is this one. Gaining knowledge of and leverage from this relationship may result in more efficient and long-lasting weight reduction.

2. Emotional Well-Being and Control of Weight:
    Our food and exercise habits are directly influenced by our mental health. For instance, stress might cause emotional eating and a predilection for comfort foods heavy in calories. On the other hand, adopting a positive outlook might inspire us to lead active lives and make better decisions. Deep breathing exercises and other

mindfulness techniques may help reduce stress and foster a more mindful connection with eating.

3. Psychological Wellness and Physical Well-Being:
Our emotional and bodily states are intricately linked. Anxiety and despair are examples of negative emotions that may upset the hormonal balance and cause weight gain or make it harder to lose weight. Positive feelings, on the other hand, may promote weight reduction by accelerating metabolic processes. Particularly helpful are somatic exercises, which alleviate stress and enhance emotional health.

4. The Awareness Role:
A vital element of the mind-body link is awareness. By increasing our awareness of our emotions, hunger signals, and physical sensations, we may make well-informed choices that support our weight reduction objectives. Engaging in somatic activities helps us become more aware of our bodies and learn how to listen to and meet their demands.

5. Scenarios and Objective Establishment:
A useful technique that makes use of the mind-body link is visualization. Through the process of picturing our goals like a fitter, healthier body we may form an internal picture that directs our behavior. Setting goals and visualizing them together gives us a clear road map for

our weight reduction journey and keeps us focused on our goals.

6. Influence of One's Own Perception:
Our behavior and self-care routines are influenced by our self-perception. Neglect and unhealthy behaviors may result from a poor self-image, while a good self-image promotes self-compassion and healthy habits. Somatic exercises help people feel good about their bodies by making them feel accomplished and appreciative of their bodies.

7. Combining the Mental and Physical Domains:
Being conscious and present during meals and exercise is crucial for incorporating the mind-body link into weight reduction.
   - Practice somatic activities to improve emotional control and bodily awareness.
   - To help you stay motivated, use visualization and positive affirmations.
   - Develop self-compassion and a good self-image.

A key component of weight reduction that transcends diet and exercise regimens is the mind-body link. It includes our emotional well-being, mental condition, and sense of self. We may strengthen this bond by adopting somatic activities and mindfulness exercises, which will result in a more comprehensive and fruitful approach to weight reduction.

11 Somatic Exercises For Weight Loss

How Physical Activity Can Help With Weight Loss

A kind of focused movement called somatic exercises may be a game-changer when it comes to losing weight. Somatic exercises include an emphasis on interior awareness, soft movements, and the mind-body connection, in contrast to traditional workouts that often emphasize high intensity and repetition. Here's how these workouts may help you lose weight:

1. Stress Reduction: Prolonged stress causes the hormone cortisol, which enhances hunger and fat storage, to be released, which may result in weight gain. By encouraging relaxation and lowering cortisol levels in the body, somatic activities assist manage stress and support weight management.

2. Improved Metabolism: By increasing blood circulation and tissue oxygenation, these activities improve metabolic function. The body's systems operating at a higher efficiency may accelerate metabolism and improve calorie burning.

3. Enhanced Body Awareness: Through somatic activities, people may become more aware of their bodies, which improves their ability to interpret signs related to hunger and fullness. This knowledge may promote better eating practices and stop overindulging in food.

4. Muscle Engagement: Somatic activities engage muscles deeper than regular workouts because they emphasize the quality of

movement. Despite the fact that the actions are often slow and methodical, this deep muscle activation may improve muscular tone and hasten fat loss.

5. Reduced Muscle Tension: An overly tense body may impede physical activity and promote a sedentary lifestyle by causing bad posture and ineffective movement patterns. It becomes simpler to participate in regular exercise and everyday activities when this tension is released via somatic exercises.

6. Emotional Release: A lot of the time, emotional reasons lead to weight gain. By giving pent-up emotions a way to be let out, somatic exercises may help prevent emotional eating and promote a more balanced relationship with food.

7. Mindful Movement: Practicing mindful movement may change the way you feel about working out. It promotes a thoughtful attitude to exercise, which enhances its enjoyment and sustainability when included into a weight reduction program.

8. Increased Flexibility and movement: The capacity to engage in a range of physical activities advances along with improvements in flexibility and movement. This may result in an overall rise in daily energy expenditure, which helps with weight reduction.

9. Hormonal Balance: Practicing somatics helps support the proper balance of hormones linked to hunger, fullness, and

controlling weight. These workouts may have a good impact on hormonal health by lowering stress and increasing sleep quality.

10. Integration with Daily Life: Somatic exercises provide regular, low-impact physical activity that promotes weight reduction without the need for strenuous, time-consuming workouts since they can be included into everyday activities.

Somatic exercises provide a comprehensive approach to weight loss, addressing not only the physical but also the mental and emotional elements of weight loss. This all-encompassing strategy may provide more significant and long-lasting outcomes, enabling weight reduction to become a more joyful and integrated aspect of a person's daily.

CHAPTER 2: The Somatic Movement Principles

Somatic movement is based on body awareness and emphasizes thoughtful movements to improve the mind-body connection and alleviate stress. It entails slow, deliberate motions that enhance proprioception, retrain the nervous system, and promote overall wellbeing. By encouraging people to investigate and comprehend their bodily experiences, this technique may help people move more fluidly and achieve a healthy balance between their mental and physical well-being.

Examining Motor Amnesia with Sensory

The term "sensory motor amnesia" (SMA) was developed to characterize a condition in which regular muscle patterns cause the body to forget how to move pleasantly and effectively. Understanding this phenomena is essential to realizing how effective somatic workouts are in enhancing physical function and promoting weight reduction.

1. The SMA Nature-
   SMA is the result of muscles losing their voluntary control due to persistent tightness. Numerous things, including stress, wounds, repeated motions, and mental trauma, may cause this. The impacted muscles continue to contract,

using up energy and decreasing the body's general effectiveness.

2. Repercussions of SMA:
   The effects of SMA are extensive. Reduced mobility, persistent discomfort, bad posture, and ineffective movement patterns might result from it. Because the body is not operating at its best, these problems might hinder attempts to reduce weight in addition to having an impact on physical health.

3. Identifying SMA:
   Because SMA develops gradually, it is sometimes overlooked. A technique of self-awareness and movement investigation is used to diagnose it. People with SMA may feel that certain motions are uncomfortable or limited, suggesting the body parts that are impacted.

4. Using Somatic Exercises to Treat SMA:
   The purpose of somatic workouts is to particularly address SMA. They entail deliberate, gradual motions that facilitate the restoration of neural and muscular connection. People may recover control and ease their involuntary tension by actively clenching and then gently releasing the tense muscles.

Advantages of Treating SMA

- Improved Movement: When SMA is treated, people have better mobility and utilize their muscles more effectively.
- Pain Relief: As their muscles relax and revert to their original condition, many patients report feeling a considerable reduction in pain.
- Enhanced Body Awareness: Breaking free from SMA helps people become more aware of their bodies, which enables them to identify and avoid harmful habits in the future.
- Weight reduction Support: The body can perform physical activities more efficiently when muscle function is enhanced and stress is decreased, which aids in weight reduction efforts.

Including Somatic Sensitivity:

It is essential to incorporate somatic awareness into everyday life in order to get the full benefits of somatic exercises. This entails continuously observing the body's cues and making the proper movement decisions in response. This exercise has the potential to significantly alter the way the body feels and moves over time, improving general health and helping with weight control.

Regaining the body's natural ability to move may be achieved by investigating and treating Sensory Motor Amnesia via somatic exercises. It is a crucial step for anybody trying to support their weight reduction objectives and improve their physical well-being.

17 Somatic Exercises For Weight Loss

Releasing Tension in Chronic Muscles

Many people suffer from chronic muscular tension, which often results in pain, discomfort, and restricted movement. Numerous things, such as stress, bad posture, repeated actions, or unresolved emotional difficulties, might contribute to it. It's critical to release this stress for your general health as well as to help you lose weight and perform better during exercise.

Comprehending Persistent Muscle Tension

When the body's normal reaction to stresses, which is the tightening of muscles, does not completely relax, muscular tension may become chronic. This may eventually cause a condition where muscles are stuck in a semi-contracted position, which hurts and causes stiffness. Additionally, this ongoing strain may lead to a bodily misalignment that impairs balance and movement efficiency.

The Nervous System's Function

Muscle tension is mostly caused by the neurological system. The sympathetic nervous system triggers the "fight or flight" reaction in response to stress, which results in tense muscles. The "rest and digest" response should ideally be triggered by the parasympathetic nervous system to bring the muscles back to a relaxed condition. On the other hand, long-term stress may upset this equilibrium and cause persistent muscular tension.

Physical Activities to Release Tension

For the purpose of relieving chronic muscular tension, somatic exercises are very beneficial. These workouts emphasize deliberate, slow motions that promote muscular relaxation. Somatic exercises assist in resetting the muscle length and retraining the nervous system to relieve tension by deliberately contracting and then gently releasing the muscles.

Inhalation Methods

One of the most important steps in relieving muscular tension is proper breathing. The parasympathetic nervous system is triggered by deep, diaphragmatic breathing, which facilitates relaxation and the release of stress. Breathing exercises are often used in somatic exercises to increase their efficacy.

Mindfulness and Body Scanning

As a mindfulness exercise, body scanning entails focusing on various body regions and identifying any tense spots. Combining this practice with somatic movements might help target and release certain muscles.

Advantages of Stress Reduction

There are many advantages to releasing persistent muscular tension:

- Pain Relief: Pain and discomfort often subside when muscles relax.
- Better Posture: Better alignment and posture may be attributed to relaxed muscles.

- Increased Mobility: As muscles relax, range of motion and flexibility may increase.
- Enhanced Exercise Performance: Exercise becomes more efficient and pleasurable when there is less tension in the body, which allows for greater range of motion.
- Stress Reduction: Releasing tension might help you feel less stressed and more at peace.
- Support for Weight reduction: A calm body is better able to do physical activities, which helps with weight reduction.

Including Stress Reduction in Everyday Activities

It is crucial to integrate somatic exercises and mindfulness practices into your daily routine in order to sustain the advantages of tension release. Frequent practice may promote continued health and weight control, as well as assist stop stress from building up again.

A comprehensive strategy for weight reduction and overall health must include the release of chronic muscular tension. People may get a more at ease, balanced, and useful body via somatic practices, breathing exercises, and mindfulness, which opens the door to a more active and healthful way of living.

Awareness's Function in Movement

The conscious notice and comprehension of one's own body's movements in space is known as awareness in movement. It is an essential component of somatic workouts and is helpful for promoting weight reduction, strengthening physical health, and increasing movement efficiency.

Developing Intentional Movement

Cultivating attentive movement is the foundation of somatic exercises. This is being acutely aware of the feelings that accompany physical exertion, such as the body's equilibrium, breathing rhythm, and the sense of muscles tightening and relaxing. People who are completely present while moving might become more aware of their automatic behaviors and modify them to move more efficiently.

The Advantages of Being Aware of Movement
Enhanced awareness of movement has several advantages:
- Injury Prevention: People may prevent injuries by avoiding actions that put their bodies in danger.
- Enhanced Coordination: Sharper motions result from increased awareness, which enhances control and coordination.
- Enhanced Learning: People pick up new exercises and abilities more quickly and precisely when they are conscious of their motions.
- Better Efficiency: Using muscles more effectively minimizes needless effort and weariness when movement is done with awareness.

- Deeper Relaxation: People may intentionally relax their muscles and relieve stress as they become more cognizant of their tension patterns.

Weight Loss and Awareness

Especially when it comes to weight reduction, movement awareness is crucial. It permits people to:
- Identify and Change behaviors: Being aware of and taking action against movement behaviors, such sedentary behavior or ineffective exercise routines, may help prevent weight gain.
- Optimize exercises: By making sure that every action is done with thought and purpose, exercises may be improved for better outcomes.
- Connect with the Body: A good body image and a better relationship with food and exercise may result from cultivating a strong connection with the body.

Real-World Uses

The following are some ways that people may put the awareness in movement principle into practice
- Practice Somatic Exercises: Regularly do somatic exercises to develop body awareness and movement quality.
- Employ Body Scanning: Before and after a workout, check your body to identify any tense or uncomfortable spots.

- Consider Movement: Consider the sensations that the body has both during and after movement, taking note of any trends or potential improvement areas.

Including Awareness in Everyday Activities

To incorporate awareness into everyday life, one must deliberately strive to pay attention to the way one's body moves whether sitting, standing, walking, or doing other tasks. This continuous practice may promote weight reduction and general well-being by fostering a more thoughtful and health-conscious lifestyle.

The importance of movement awareness is a fundamental aspect of somatic exercises and an essential step on the path to a more balanced, healthier lifestyle. People may fully use their physical potential and achieve better mobility, weight management, and overall health by cultivating this awareness.

CHAPTER 3: Introduction to Somatic Exercises

Establishing a peaceful space and a dedication to mindful practice are the first steps in starting somatic exercises. Begin with simple motions, paying attention to your breath and your body's feelings. Increase the complexity of the workouts progressively while keeping your attention within. By improving mobility, releasing tension, and enhancing body awareness, this method will provide a strong basis for your somatic journey and weight reduction objectives.

Setting Up Your Environment and Attitude

You should set up your physical environment and mental condition before doing any somatic workouts. Setting up a setting that supports mindfulness and productive practice requires some preparation.

1. Building a Friendly Environment-
Your physical surroundings need to be a haven for mobility and introspection. Here's how to get ready for it:
-Select a Calm Area: Locate a quiet area where you can be alone. It may be a particular room in your house or a remote area in the outdoors.

2. Garden Comfort: There should be enough space for movement and a pleasant atmosphere. For floor workouts, you may add cushioning with a soft mat or carpet.

3. Reduce Interruptions: Clear your area of any clutter and any distractions. Dimming bright lighting and shutting off electronics are two examples of this.

4. Determine the Scene: To create a soothing ambiance, think about using incense, candles, or soft lighting. Sounds of nature or soft background music may also improve the experience.

Developing the Appropriate Mentality

The way you mentally prepare matters as much as the actual location. Here's how to adopt the appropriate frame of mind:

- Assigning Intentions: Make an intention at the start of every session. During the exercises, it might be to just be present or to relieve stress or to become more aware of one's body.

- Mindfulness Practice: To center oneself, spend a few minutes practicing mindfulness or meditation. Let go of other concerns and concentrate on your breathing.

- Take Courage: It takes time to do somatic exercises. Treat them with kindness as you learn from them, and don't anticipate instant results.

- Remain Open: Throughout your exercise, be receptive to the feelings and experiences that surface. You may learn something new about your body with every action.

Mixing Mentality and Space

You create the best atmosphere for somatic activities when your space and mentality work together harmoniously. You can completely participate in the exercises with this preparation, which guarantees that you will get the most out of your practice. It's important to really connect with your body and let the transformational force of somatic exercises do its magic, rather than merely following the steps.

In conclusion, setting up your environment and mentality is essential before starting any somatic workouts. You may complement your weight reduction and health objectives with a fulfilling and meaningful somatic experience by setting up a calm atmosphere and practicing mindfulness.

Safety Advice and Pointers

Safety should always come first when doing somatic exercises for weight reduction or any other reason. The following are crucial pointers and things to think about to make sure your practice is safe and efficient:

1. Consult a Professional: Speak with a healthcare physician or a qualified somatic exercise coach before to beginning any new fitness program, particularly if you already have health issues.

2. Start Slowly: If you're unfamiliar with somatic exercises, start with simple motions and work your way up to more complicated ones as your body adjusts.

3. Listen to Your Body: Throughout the exercises, pay special attention to how your body feels. If you feel pain or discomfort, pause and reconsider how you are going about things.

4. Create a Safe Space: Make sure that there are no risks or impediments in your practicing space that might lead to harm. Make use of a mat or other soft surface to provide comfort and support.

5. Remain Hydrated: To ensure that your body is properly hydrated and performing at its best, drink water before to, during, and after your practice.

6. Wear Appropriate Clothing: Decide on apparel that is both comfortable and permits unhindered mobility during your exercise.

7. Pay Attention to Form: In somatic exercises, proper form is essential. Repetitions should be performed with proper form in smaller sets rather than in larger ones to avoid damage.

8. Use Props if Needed: When learning new exercises, in particular, props like chairs, blocks, or straps may assist you maintain alignment and balance.

9. Avoid Overexertion: Pushing yourself to the maximum is not the point of somatic exercises. They include light, deliberate motions. Refrain from exerting too much energy as this may result in strained muscles.

10. Incorporate Rest: Give yourself enough time in between sessions to recuperate. The goal of somatic workouts is quality over quantity.

11. Mindful Breathing: Throughout exercises, always breathe thoughtfully and never hold your breath. Breathing correctly keeps the muscles oxygenated and helps to avoid vertigo.

12. Regular Practice: In somatic exercises, consistency is essential. Practice on a regular basis will improve performance and lower the chance of injury.

13. Adapt as Needed: Adjust workouts to your own requirements and physical constraints. Somatic movement cannot be approached in a one-size-fits-all manner.

14. Cool Down: After your practice, give yourself a moment to relax and let your body and heart rate to return to normal.

You may minimize the danger of damage and yet get the full advantages of somatic workouts by paying attention to these safety recommendations and considerations. Recall that somatic practice aims to improve your general well-being and help you develop a stronger connection with your body, all while safely and sustainably assisting in your weight reduction journey.

Required Gear & Clothes

The goal of somatic exercise is to promote body awareness and ease of movement by emphasizing comfort and usefulness. The following list of necessities includes both clothing and equipment:

- Meeting Place for Comfort and Mobility Apparel: Don loose, comfortable garments that don't impede your range of motion. Natural textiles that breathe well, like cotton or bamboo, may assist control body temperature.
- Footwear: To improve proprioception the body's awareness of its location in spacee somatic activities are usually done barefoot. Grip-bottom socks may provide warmth when needed without compromising feeling.

Support and Alignment Equipment
1. Exercise Mat: A high-quality mat cushions floor workouts and aids in creating personal space. Select a mat that is both hard enough to keep your balance and thick enough to support your joints.
2. Supportive Props: For those with restricted flexibility or certain medical problems, tools like as folded blankets, yoga blocks, or bolsters may be used to support the body during certain exercises.

3. Resistance Bands: Although not necessary, resistance bands may increase the difficulty of certain somatic exercises and aid in the development of strength and awareness in the targeted muscle regions.

Practice-Improving Tools

1. Mirrors: Having a mirror in your area of practice may aid with self-observation by enabling you to assess your alignment and form throughout exercises.

2. Diary: Managing your weight loss journey and strengthening your somatic practice may both benefit from keeping a diary in which you record your experiences, sensations, and progress.

3. Timer or App: To ensure that you remain present and don't worry about time, use a basic timer or a specialized app to measure the length of your practice.

Creating an Inviting Atmosphere

- Music or Soundscapes: Calm ambient sounds or soothing background music might improve the somatic experience.
- Aromatherapy: To stimulate your sense of smell and assist create a calming atmosphere, think about using scented candles or essential oils.

Safety and Hygiene

1. Cleanliness: If you're practicing in a communal area, make sure your equipment is sanitary and clean. Bacteria and smells may be avoided by routinely cleaning your mat and props.

2. Personal Towel: Keep a little towel nearby to control sweat and make sure your hands and feet are dry for safety.

You can make your somatic workout regimen more pleasurable and successful by setting up a practice space that supports it with the appropriate gear and clothes. This will help you on your path to weight reduction and wellbeing. It is important to keep in mind that selecting objects that improve your comfort and sense of connection to your body will enable you to fully experience the transformational potential of somatic movement.

CHAPTER 4: Simple Somatic Motions

The mind and body may be reconnected via somatic exercises, which are soft and aware. They include deliberate, calm movements that alleviate stress and increase self-awareness. Retraining the nervous system, increasing flexibility, and reestablishing natural movement patterns are the main goals of basic somatic movements. These fundamental exercises are essential for fostering body awareness and may be used as a springboard for more complex somatic approaches to improved health and weight reduction.

The Series on Cat Stretching

A basic series of somatic exercises called the Cat Stretch Series is intended to alleviate chronic muscular tension and stimulate the body's sensory-motor system. This series may be a potent tool for weight reduction and enhancing general well-being, and it is especially beneficial for those who are just starting out with somatic activities.

History and Thought
The organic stretching motions seen in cats serve as the model for the Cat Stretch Series. These animals are renowned for their elegance and fluidity, often stretching in an innate way to

maintain their agility. In a similar vein, the Cat Stretch Series invites people to rediscover their natural ability to move effortlessly.

Parts of the Stretch Series for Cats

The series comprises of many motions that focus on various body parts:

1. Arch and Flatten: This exercise is breathing with the back softly arched upwards like a cat, then exhaling with the back slowly flattened. It facilitates improved flexibility and the elimination of spinal stress.

2. Back Lift: The practitioner engages the back muscles and improves spinal health by elevating the head, chest, and opposing leg while the patient is face down.

3. Side Bend: The body is bent sideways while sitting or standing, which lengthens the lateral muscles and increases the flexibility of the spine from side to side.

4.Diagonal Arch: This technique includes increasing coordination, extending and using the oblique muscles, and arching the back diagonally.

Advantages of the Cat Stretch Series

1. Improved Body Awareness: Engaging in these exercises promotes proprioception and makes people more aware of their bodies' demands and capacities.

2. Stress Relief: The stretches' deliberate and rhythmic style encourages relaxation and may aid in reducing stress, which is often a barrier to weight reduction.

33 Somatic Exercises For Weight Loss

3. Improved Posture: By strengthening the core muscles and straightening the spine, regular practice helps improve posture.
4. Increased Flexibility: By gradually stretching the muscles, the range of motion and flexibility are increased.
5. Muscle Tone: By doing these exercises, you can tone and shape your body, which will help you lose weight.

Adding the Cat Stretch Series to Your Daily Schedule

Include the Cat Stretch Series in your regular routine to start reaping its advantages. Start small, a few minutes a day, and as your body adjusts, gradually extend the time. It's crucial to move deliberately and gently, paying more attention to your body's feelings than its range of motion.

Any somatic exercise regimen would benefit from the inclusion of the Cat Stretch Series, especially those that aim to lose weight. You may improve your relationship with your body, relieve stress, and cultivate a feeling of wellbeing that complements your health objectives by doing these exercises on a daily basis. To ensure a fun and safe practice, pay attention to your body and modify the motions to your comfort level.

Pelvic Clock Workout

A fundamental somatic exercise that encourages awareness and control of the pelvic area is the Pelvic Clock Exercise. Its name comes from the idea that the pelvis may be seen as the face of a clock, with the pubic bone standing in for six o'clock and the navel for twelve. This exercise may be very useful for those who want to lose weight and have an active lifestyle since it helps to improve pelvic mobility, align the spine, and release lower back strain.

Exercise Procedure for the Pelvic Clock

1. -Beginning Position: Lay flat on your back with your feet flat on the ground and your knees bent. You want your arms to be at ease at your sides.

2. Create a Clock Image: Envision the edge of your pelvis as the face of a clock. 12 o'clock is the position at your navel, and 6 o'clock is the point immediately across from it at the base of your spine. Three and nine are the hip bones.

3. Shift to 12 and 6: Flatten your lower back into the floor by gently tilting your pelvis towards your navel to shift the 12 o'clock point downward. Next, raise your lower back and shift the point at six o'clock higher by tilting your pelvis in the direction of your feet.

4. Move to 3 and 9: Make a side-to-side rocking motion by shifting your weight to move your pelvis towards one hip bone (3 o'clock) and then the other hip bone (9 o'clock).

5. Circular Motion: Use these motions in combination to spin your pelvis in a clockwise and counterclockwise circle. Continue to move in a controlled, fluid manner.

Pelvic Clock Exercise Benefits
- Spinal Alignment: This workout promotes healthy spine alignment, which helps reduce back discomfort and improve posture.
- Core Engagement: The mild rotation and tilting work the core muscles, which help to tone the abdominal region and are vital for stability.
- Strengthening of the Pelvic Floor: The Pelvic Clock Exercise tones the muscles supporting the internal organs and adds to the overall strength of the core.
- Flexibility: Consistent practice improves hip and lower back flexibility, which improves mobility and lowers the chance of injury when engaging in other activities.
- Mind-Body Connection: By emphasizing pelvic mobility, one may improve one's mind-body connection, which in turn helps one relax and reduce stress.

Including the Pelvic Clock in Your Daily Activities
Practice the Pelvic Clock Exercise every day, preferably in the morning or before doing any other physical activity, to make it a part of your routine. It may be done on its own to maintain pelvic health or as a warm-up to get your body ready for more strenuous activity.

A simple but effective technique for anybody trying to enhance their somatic awareness and physical health is the Pelvic Clock Exercise. Regularly engaging in this exercise can help you achieve your fitness and weight reduction objectives by strengthening your core, improving your pelvic mobility, and strengthening your connection with your body. Keep in mind to walk slowly and pay attention to your body so that the exercise may be a restorative and relaxing experience.

The Exercise with Flowers

The Flower Exercise is a somatic practice that emphasizes the body's slow opening and shutting in response to light, much like a flower does. The goal of this exercise is to foster a feeling of physical and emotional expansion and contraction as well as a greater awareness of the body's inherent rhythms.

How to Complete the Flower Task
1. Beginning Position: Take a comfortable seat in a chair with your feet flat on the floor or on the floor with your legs crossed. Place your hands on your thighs or knees.
2. Inhale and Open: Lean your arms gently over your head, opening your chest and lengthening your spine as you take a deep breath. Visualize your body blossoming like a flower.
3. Exhale and Close: Draw your body inward, lowering your arms and rounding your spine slowly, as if you were a flower shutting its petals at nightfall.
4. Repeat: Keep moving in a smooth manner while timing the opening and shutting of your body with your breath.

Advantages of the Flower Practice

- Enhanced Breath Control: This exercise promotes diaphragmatic breathing, which may lower stress levels and increase oxygenation.
- Increased Spinal Mobility: The exercise encourages the spine to become more flexible, which may reduce back discomfort and improve posture.
- Emotional Release: Letting go of emotional stress and accepting good energy may be symbolized by the opening and closing gestures.
- Mindfulness: By encouraging a contemplative state, the Flower Exercise improves mindfulness and awareness of the present moment.
- Core Strengthening: Your core muscles contract as you move your arms and correct your posture, which strengthens your midsection.

Adding the Flower Exercise to Your Daily Schedule

Although the Flower Exercise may be done at any time of day, it could be particularly helpful to do it in the morning to help the body awaken or in the evening to help with relaxation. It may be a stand-alone exercise or a component of a more extensive somatic regimen.

The Flower Exercise encompasses the fundamentals of somatic movement and is a simple but deep exercise. You may get physical advantages from increased flexibility and core strength as well as mental benefits from stress alleviation and emotional balance by doing this exercise on a regular basis. It's an adaptable exercise that may help you lose weight by strengthening your connection with your body and your body's natural intelligence. Always remember to take a patient and moderate approach to the exercise, letting your body lead you through the moves.

CHAPTER 5: Moderate Somatic Activities

Building on foundational methods, intermediate somatic movements provide more difficult exercises that improve muscle control and body awareness. These exercises often entail strengthening flexibility, testing balance, and integrating the upper and lower bodies. Regular practice supports a comprehensive approach to health and weight control by promoting better posture, lower stress levels, and a greater connection between the mind and body.

The Series of Side Bends

An intermediate series of somatic exercises, the Side Bend Series targets the lateral flexion of the spine. These exercises aim to improve general body alignment, strengthen the oblique muscles, and increase flexibility. People who practice the Side Bend Series may improve their body's sense of symmetry and balance, which is especially advantageous for those who want to use mindful movement to support their weight reduction efforts.

How to Execute It
1. Starting Position: Either sit comfortably with your back straight or stand with your feet hip-width apart.

2. Lateral Flexion: With your hips in line, raise one arm over your head and slowly bend your body to the other side. Along the side of your body, feel the stretch.

3. Dynamic Movement: Bend again on the other side, then slowly return to the beginning position. Breathe as you move; take a breath as you raise your arm and release it when you bend.

4. Progression: Using a modest weight in the raised hand, you may gradually add resistance or extend the range of motion as you gain familiarity with the exercise.

The Side Bend Series' advantages

- Spinal Health: By making the vertebrae more flexible and less rigid, these exercises help to maintain the health of the spine.
- Core Strengthening: The bends work the oblique muscles, which helps to stabilize and build the lower back.
- Better Posture: By equally strengthening the muscles on both sides of the body, regular exercise helps improve posture.
- Enhanced Breathing: Intercostal muscle stretching may increase lung capacity and breathing effectiveness.
- Stress Relief: Concentrated breathing and the rhythmic motions may have a relaxing impact on the neurological system.

Including the Side Bend Series in Your Daily Activities

You may perform the Side Bend Series as a warm-up before more strenuous physical activity, or you can add it into your regular somatic exercises. In order to relax after a demanding day, it may also be used as a restorative therapy.

With advantages for the body and mind, the Side Bend Series is a great complement to any somatic workout regimen. You may assist your weight reduction objectives and meet your body's demand for harmonic, balanced movement by including these motions into your regimen. To ensure a safe and productive practice, pay attention to your body's signals and modify the strength of the bends to suit your comfort level.

The Walking Activity
An intermediate somatic exercise, the walking exercise aims to integrate the complete body in a thoughtful and natural manner. This workout, in contrast to ordinary walking, places an emphasis on the caliber of each step, body alignment, and awareness of movement patterns. It's a great exercise for anyone who want a low-impact, full-body movement to support their weight reduction goals.

How to Do It
1. Starting Position: Place your arms at your sides in a comfortable manner, look ahead, and stand with your feet hip-width apart.
2. Mindful Steps: Take a few leisurely steps at first, focusing entirely on how each foot feels on the ground. Observe how your weight shifts from your heel to your toes.

3. Breath Coordination: Sync your breathing with your steps by taking one breath for every step and releasing air after that same number of steps. This promotes calm and aids in keeping the tempo regular.

4. Arm Movement: Let your arms swing organically in sync with your gait. To improve balance and the cross-body connection, the opposing arm and leg should move in unison.

5. Posture Awareness: Maintain an extended spine, relaxed shoulders, and a strong core. This alignment facilitates effective mobility and lessens physical stress on the body.

Benefits

1. Cardiovascular Health: This workout improves cardiovascular fitness without the strain of high-impact exercises by gradually raising heart rate.

2.Muscle Engagement: Walking works the arms, legs, and core, among other muscle groups, offering a whole body exercise.

3.Mental Clarity: The contemplative nature of mindful walking helps enhance attention, ease anxiety, and cleanse the mind.

4.Weight reduction: By gradually and sustainably raising daily calorie expenditure, regular practice may aid in weight reduction.

5.Enhanced Coordination: By emphasizing cross-body movement patterns, neuromuscular control and coordination are improved.

Adding the Walking Exercise to Your Daily Schedule

There are many methods to include the Walking Exercise into your everyday routine:

1. As a Warm-Up: Do this to get your body ready for more strenuous activity.

2. As a Stand-Alone Practice: Set aside a certain period of time, such an evening or a work break, for mindful walking.

-Incorporated into Daily Tasks: Whether you're at home, the office, or doing errands, walk mindfully throughout the day.

A flexible and easily accessible somatic exercise, walking has several advantages for mental and physical well-being. Your weight reduction program may benefit from a comprehensive approach to fitness that nourishes the body and soothes the mind by using this workout. Recall to approach the exercise with care and focus, letting your body's natural rhythm dictate how you move.

The Modal Inversion

An intermediate somatic exercise, the Somatic Twist uses a sequence of rotating motions to work the pelvic muscles, spine, and core. This activity may help with weight reduction and general well-being since it strengthens and stretches the torso, supports spinal health, and facilitates digestion.

How to Execute It

1. Starting Position: Either sit on a chair with your feet flat on the floor or sit on the floor with your legs out in front of you.

2. Start the Twist: Support yourself with one hand behind your back. Reach over to the outside of your opposing leg or knee with your other hand.

3. Gentle Rotation: Maintaining your hips square and your spine extended, slowly rotate your torso towards the back hand as you exhale.

4. Hold and Release: Hold the pose for a few breaths, paying attention to how your spine stretches and rotates. Take a breath to let go and go back to where you were.

5. Repeat on the Other Side: To keep your body balanced, repeat the twist on the other side.

Benefits

1. Spinal Decompression: By allowing the vertebrae to loosen up and decompress, pressure and tension in the spine are reduced.

2. Core Activation: The twist strengthens the core, which is necessary for proper posture and movement, by contracting the abdominal and oblique muscles.

3. Enhanced Digestion: The abdominal organs' massaging action may improve digestion and support the body's detoxification procedures.

4. Increased Flexibility: By regularly doing the Somatic Twist, you may improve your mobility by being more flexible in your torso and spine.

5. Mind-Body Coordination: By requiring concentration and coordination, this exercise enhances general body awareness and neuromuscular communication.

Adding The Somatic Twist to Your Daily Schedule

You may include the Somatic Twist into your everyday workout regimen as a stand-alone movement or as a component of a somatic sequence. It works especially well to re-energize the body and mind after a time of sitting or inactivity.

For people who practice somatics, the Somatic Twist is a flexible workout with several advantages. You may benefit from a stronger, more flexible spine, a strong core, and a closer relationship with your body's natural rhythms by including this exercise into your regimen. As with any somatic exercises, keep in mind to move mindfully and with consideration for your body's limitations so that the twist may serve as a strengthening and restorative activity.

CHAPTER 6: Higher Level Somatic Activities

Complex exercises known as advanced somatic movements expand on the concepts of body awareness, mindfulness, and purposeful movement learned in basic and intermediate practices. With the aim of pushing the body and mind to new limits, these exercises aim to increase strength, flexibility, and neuromuscular coordination. They are perfect for anyone who are wanting to assist their weight reduction journey and improve their physical skills and have a strong basis in somatic exercises.

Features of Complex Somatic Movements
- Complexity: Since these exercises often include many movement patterns, they call for a higher level of focus and control.
- Intensity: More complex motions may include more forceful and dynamic movements, all the while maintaining a conscious execution focus.
- Integration: Complex techniques include the whole body, necessitating synchronization between various body regions and muscle groups.
- Accuracy: To ensure safety and efficacy, these motions need a high degree of accuracy.

Advanced Somatic Movement Examples

1. Cross-Patterning Marches: This exercise requires you to simultaneously elevate your opposing arm and leg while marching while keeping your alignment and balance.

2. Somatic Sun Salutations: An elegant sequence of motions that fuse the sun salutations of classical yoga with the awareness of the body, emphasizing the seamless flow between positions.

3. Dynamic Planks: To strengthen your core and stability, try plank variants that include arm reaches, leg lifts, or side planks.

4. Rotational Lunges: To strengthen the obliques and increase rotational mobility, twist your lunges.

Benefits

- Improved Physical Fitness: These workouts may increase cardiovascular health, strength, and endurance.

- Better Understanding of Your Body: The intricacy of the motions encourages a more thorough comprehension of your body's potential and limitations.

- Improved Movement Quality: Consistent practice helps improve movement patterns, which facilitates and expedites daily tasks.

- Weight Loss Support: Higher calorie burn and muscle growth may result from advanced motions' greater physical demands.

Adding Complex Somatic Exercises to Your Daily Schedule
Take into consideration the following while adding advanced somatic motions to your program in a healthy manner:

1. Gradual Progression: Prior to undertaking difficult workouts, make sure you have mastered basic and intermediate moves.

2. Warm-Up: To get your muscles and joints ready for the higher demands, always start with a complete warm-up.

3. Expert Counseling: To correctly acquire advanced methods, working with a somatic exercise practitioner might be advantageous.

4. Pay Attention to Your Body: To prevent overdoing it or getting hurt, pay careful attention to how your body reacts to the exercises and make any adjustments.

For individuals who want to go deeper into their somatic experience, advanced somatic movements provide a rich and satisfying exercise. You may experience an enhanced feeling of physical and mental well-being by participating in these activities, which can be a beneficial tool in your weight reduction and overall health journey. Treat these advanced motions with attention, patience, and respect for your body's knowledge, as you would any somatic exercise.

The series of helicopters

The fundamental and intermediate somatic exercise routines culminate in advanced somatic movements. These motions are distinguished by their intricacy and the profound degree of bodily awareness they need. They are made to put the body's movement patterns to the test, improve proprioception, and achieve a deeper degree of mind-body integration.

Features of Complex Somatic Movements

1. Complexity: Complex motions often need coordination and focus since they include numerous planes of motion.

2 Precision: To perform these workouts correctly, muscle groups must be precisely controlled.

3. Integration: For comprehensive benefits, they need the integration of the whole body, working several muscle groups at once.

Advanced Somatic Movement Examples

1. Cross-Patterning Sequences: Balance and coordination-testing movements in which opposing limbs move in unison.

2. Dynamic Reaching: Reaching exercises that strengthen the core and increase flexibility while increasing the body's range of motion.

3. Rotational Discs: Spinal health and agility are promoted by movements that rotate the body or limbs around an axis.

4. Balance Challenges: Activities that measure your ability to maintain balance, such standing on one leg while moving your upper body.

The advantages of advanced somatic movements include improved control over posture and movement, or Enhanced Motor Control

- Increased Strength and Flexibility: The growth of muscles that are more resilient and capable of supporting a healthy weight.

- Stress Reduction: Advanced somatic exercises include a meditative component that helps lessen stress and the weight gain that comes with it.
- Improved Athletic Performance: These motions provide athletes more agility and coordination, which is beneficial.

Adding Complex Somatic Exercises to Your Daily Schedule
It's crucial to -Build a Strong Foundation- in order to properly include advanced somatic movements into your practice. Make sure you are comfortable with basic and intermediate somatic exercises before moving on.
1. Warm-Up Properly: To get your body ready for the demands of advanced motions, warm up thoroughly.
2. Practice Often: To become proficient in these exercises and experience their advantages, regular practice is essential.
3. Remain Conscious: Recognize your body's limitations at all times and refrain from pushing yourself beyond discomfort or pain.

More complex somatic exercises provide a way to strengthen the link between the mind and body, which may enhance physical well-being and help with weight control. They provide as evidence of the body's amazing range of motion and adaptability. As with any workout, they should be performed safely and with appreciation for the body's limits and present condition.

The Bow and Arrow Exercise is a sophisticated somatic exercise that simulates the motion of drawing a bow by putting the body through a dynamic stretch. This is a great workout to strengthen the back muscles, increase shoulder flexibility, and open up the chest. It helps offset the forward hunching posture, which is especially advantageous for those who have sedentary lifestyles or spend a lot of time sitting down.

How to Complete the Exercise with Bow and Arrow
1. Starting Position: Either sit in a chair with a straight back or stand with your feet hip-width apart.
2. Arm Position: With your palms facing ahead, extend your arms out to the sides at shoulder height.
3. Drawing the Bow:With your other arm stretched like a bow, draw one hand back as if you were drawing a bowstring as you inhale. Turn your head to face the hand that is retraction.
4. Hold and Focus: As you hold the pose for a few breaths, pay attention to how your back muscles are contracting and how your chest is stretched.
5. Release and Repeat: Let out a breath and carefully raise your arms back to the beginning position. On the opposite side, repeat the motion.

Advantages of the Bow and Arrow Exercise
1. Enhanced Posture: Consistent exercise helps build stronger muscles involved in maintaining an erect posture.

2. Increased Lung Capacity: The exercise's chest expansion promotes deeper breathing, which has the potential to expand lung capacity.

3. Shoulder Health: By increasing shoulder range of motion and flexibility, the exercise helps shield the area against injury and discomfort.

4. Stress Relief: Since the chest opening is often the site of emotional tension storage, it may help relieve stress.

5. Enhanced Focus: This exercise improves mental clarity and focus since it requires coordination.

Adding the Bow and Arrow Exercise to Your Daily Schedule
You may include this exercise into your regular somatic practice, particularly after times of inactivity or as a respite from desk job. Additionally, it may be used as a warm-up before playing sports or doing other physical exercises.

With advantages for the body and mind, the Bow and Arrow Exercise is a potent instrument in the somatic movement repertory. You may experience better posture, more flexibility, and a sensation of release in your upper body by including this exercise into your program. The practice may be both healing and energizing if you approach it with attention and respect for your body's limitations, as with other advanced somatic exercises.

The Somatic Board
The Somatic Plank is an advanced exercise that combines the body awareness and mindfulness that are essential to somatic

practices with the physical difficulty of the standard plank. This exercise improves stability and control by strengthening the core and fostering a strong mental-physical connection.

How to Perform It

1. Starting posture: Place your forearms and toes on the floor to start in the classic plank posture. Make sure your body makes a straight line from your head to your heels and that your elbows are squarely under your shoulders.

2. Engage Mindfully: Use every muscle group by actively engaging them rather than just maintaining the posture passively. Your abs should be tightened first, followed by your thighs, calves, and glutes.

3. Integrating Breath:Continue breathing deeply and rhythmically. Imagine that you are transferring energy down your spine with each exhale, strengthening and extending your posture.

4. Micro-Movements: To test your stability and increase muscular activation, start with little, controlled motions like softly rocking forward and backward or side to side.

5. Hold and Release: Take a few deep breaths while holding the plank, and then gradually lower your body to the ground. Take a break and then repeat the workout.

Somatic Plank Advantages

1. Core Strength: This exercise is great for strengthening the core, which is necessary for proper posture and balance.

2. Body Awareness: The somatic method promotes an increased awareness of the alignment and activation of the body's muscles.

3. Mental attention: The Somatic Plank helps enhance mental clarity and attention by requiring concentration.

4. Stress Reduction: Physical activity together with conscious breathing may help lower stress levels.

5. Weight Loss Aid: By raising muscle mass and metabolic rate, the Somatic Plank, a strength-building exercise, may help reduce weight.

Including The Somatic Plank in Your Daily Activities
You may include the Somatic Plank as a core-strengthening exercise in your workout program. When paired with other somatic motions in a flow from one exercise to the next, it is very beneficial.

The Somatic Plank is an effective workout that improves mental and physical health. You can assist your weight reduction objectives, strengthen your core, and increase your body awareness by doing this exercise on a daily basis. To guarantee a safe and successful practice, always remember to approach the exercise with mindfulness, honoring your body's limitations and concentrating on the quality of movement.

CHAPTER 7: Somatic Activities for Particular Requirements

Individualized somatic workouts target personal health issues and objectives. These customized motions target specific areas such as strength, flexibility, or balance and are tailored to fit different capacities and circumstances. Somatic exercises may help with recuperation, performance enhancement, and general well-being by focusing on specific demands. As such, they are an invaluable resource for anybody looking to improve their physical health and quality of life.

To Boost Harmony and Equilibrium

Physical health requires balance and coordination, which impact everyday activities as well as sporting performance. A better sense of spatial orientation, decreased risk of falls, and improved body control may all result from somatic workouts that target these regions.

Comprehending Equilibrium and Sync

Coordination is the capacity to carry out fluid, precise, and controlled motions of the body, while balance is the capacity to keep the body's center of gravity within its base of support. Both depend on the intricate interactions that occur between the vestibular system in the inner ear, the muscular system, and proprioception the body's awareness of its location and movement.

Physical Activities to Improve Balance and Coordination

1. Single-Leg Stands: Balance is improved by using the core and stabilizer muscles while standing on one leg at a time. Close your eyes or stand on an unsteady surface to make things more challenging.

2. Heel-to-Toe Walks: Replicating the "sobriety test" walk, walking in a straight line with one foot in front of the other tests balance and coordination.

3. Tai Chi Movements: By promoting mindfulness and body awareness, the slow, methodical movements of Tai Chi improve balance and coordination.

4. Balance Boards or Discs: Using balance boards or discs improves proprioceptive ability by requiring continuous microadjustments in joint position and muscle tension.

5. Dance Therapy: Dancing is a fun approach to improve balance and coordination since it contains intricate motions that call for rhythmic and motor coordination.

Advantages of Enhancing Balance and Coordination

Prevention of Injuries: Enhanced balance and coordination may help avoid falls and injuries associated with them, particularly in elderly individuals.

1. Enhanced Athletic Performance: Faster reflexes and greater agility are advantages for athletes.

2. Increased Cognitive Function: These workouts may improve cognitive skills since they need a focused mental effort.

3. Improved Posture: Proper posture helps reduce discomfort and facilitate breathing. It is facilitated by a strong feeling of balance.

Including Exercises for Balance and Coordination in Your Routine

Start with brief sessions to introduce these workouts into your regimen, then as your abilities develop, progressively increase the time. Exercises for balance and coordination should be done multiple times a week since consistency is essential.

Somatic exercises are a great way to enhance your balance and coordination while also benefiting your general health and well-being. These exercises improve mental clarity and self-assurance in movement in addition to improving physical skills. As with any fitness regimen, it's important to listen to your body and go at your own speed in order to prevent overdoing it.

To Increase Adaptability

Improving flexibility is essential to general health and fitness. It includes a variety of exercises that increase the muscles' and connective tissues' flexibility, increasing range of motion and lowering the chance of injury. This is a thorough guide on improving flexibility:

Benefits of Flexibility Training

1. Improves Range of Motion: Increasing joint range of motion with flexibility training may make it easier to carry out everyday tasks.

2. Reduces Risk of Injury: Training for flexibility may help avoid injuries that are often linked to tight, inflexible muscles by increasing the suppleness of muscular tissue.

3. Improves Athletic Performance: By enabling more forceful and accurate motions, flexibility training may help athletes perform better.

4. Alleviates Muscle Tension: Frequent flexibility exercises may aid in the reduction of soreness and tension in the muscles, encouraging rest and a reduction in stress.

Varieties of Training in Flexibility

1. Dynamic Flexibility: This entails moving body parts while progressively extending one's reach, one's pace, or both. It works best if done before to physical exercise to get the muscles ready for action.

2. Static Flexibility: This kind of stretching entails maintaining a stretch in a comfortable posture for an extended amount of time. It's advantageous to assist the body calm down and preserve muscular length after exercise.

3. Active Flexibility: Active stretching means maintaining a stretch with just the agonist muscles' power. It strengthens the muscles and enhances active range of motion.

4. Passive Flexibility: Passive stretching is holding a stretch with the assistance of an outside force, such a strap or another person.

Compared to active flexibility, it may aid in achieving a deeper stretch.

Techniques for Flexibility Training

1. Warm-Up: Warming up before an exercise helps improve blood flow to the muscles and lowers the chance of injury.

2. Breath Work: To assist relax the muscles and improve the efficiency of the stretches, include slow, deep breathing into your regimen.

3. Consistency: To observe results, do flexibility exercises on a regular basis. A few times a week, even ten minutes may have a big impact.

4. Progressive Overload: To maintain your flexibility improvements, gradually increase the length and intensity of your stretches.

Model Flexibility Schedule

1. Upper Body Stretches: Arm circles, wrist flexor stretches, tricep stretches, and shoulder rolls.

2. Lower Body Stretches: stretch your quadriceps, hamstrings, calves, and hip flexors.

3. Spine Stretches: Child's posture, spinal twists, and cat-cow stretches.

4. Complete Body Stretches: dynamic leg swings, walking lunges with a twist, and inchworms.

Safety Advice

1. Pay Attention to Your Body: Avoid pushing a stretch to the point of discomfort. Stretch till you feel a little uncomfortable, then hold it.

2. Avoid Bouncing: Bouncing during a stretch may result in tiny rips in the muscle, which may cause scarring and a reduction in flexibility.

3. Remain Hydrated: To keep the tissues supple and hydrated, drink plenty of water.

You may increase your level of fitness, improve your flexibility, and live a better quality of life by implementing these techniques into your daily routine. Never forget that anybody may benefit from flexibility exercise, regardless of age or level of fitness: it's not only for athletes. Take your time, be steady, and enjoy the process of becoming a more flexible version of yourself.

How To Develop Your Core Muscles

Maintaining balance, stability, and general health requires strengthening the core muscles. The muscles in your pelvis, lower back, hips, and abdomen are all part of your core. They are not limited to your abdominal muscles alone. Your spine and bodily motions are supported by the cooperative action of these muscles. This is a thorough approach to building stronger core muscles:

1. Advantages of Strong Core Muscles--Supports Posture: Well-developed core muscles help to maintain good posture and lessen spinal strain.

2. Improves Athletic Performance: Power, agility, and endurance are all enhanced in athletes with a strong core.

3. Prevents Injuries: By supporting the body during physical activity, a stable core guards against injuries.

4. Improves Balance and Stability: Especially for older persons, core strength is essential for balance and lowers the risk of falls.

Rectus Abdominis: Also referred to as the "abs," these muscles run vertically down the front of the abdomen. They are one of the key core muscles to target.

1. Obliques: These abdominal muscles aid in lateral and rotational movement. They are situated on the sides.

The deepest layer of the abdominal muscles, the -Transverse Abdominis-, is crucial for maintaining core stability.

2. Erector Spinae: A set of muscles that span the length of your spine and are vital to the strength of your back.

3. Glutes: An essential component of the core, these muscles provide strength and stability to the lower body.

Powerful Exercises to Strengthen Your Core

1. Planks: Use your whole core without putting too much tension on your back. For a duration of 30 to 60 seconds, maintain a plank posture.

2. Russian Twists: Bend your knees while sitting on the floor, tuck your head in slightly, and rotate your body back and forth.

3. Bird Dogs: Extend one arm and the opposing leg while starting on your hands and knees. Then, swap sides.

4. Dead Bugs: Arms extended toward the ceiling, alternately extend the opposing arm and leg while lying on your back.

5. Bridges: Lower yourself back down to the floor while lying on your back with your legs bent. Hold the pose for a moment.

Core Training Tips

1. Consistency is Key: Strengthening and preserving your core requires regular workout.

2. Quality Over Quantity: Pay more attention to the form and technique of each workout than to the quantity of reps.

3. Progressive Overload: To keep your muscles challenged, progressively raise the level of workouts.

4. Inhaling: Breathing correctly during an activity promotes greater execution and helps activate the core.

Model Core Exercise Schedule

1. Warm-Up: 5 minutes of mild cardio to get the heart pumping.

2. Connection: The circuit below should be repeated two or three times, with a 30- to 1-minute break in between each exercise:

  Planks: thirty seconds

  - 15 repetitions on each side for Russian twists

  - 10 repetitions on each side for Bird Dogs

  Dead Bugs: ten repetitions on each side

  - Bridges: fifteen repetitions

Security Warnings

1. Pay Attention to Your Body: If you experience discomfort, particularly in the lower back, pause and evaluate your form.

2. Avoid Overexertion: To avoid damage, give your muscles time to rest in between sessions.

3. Speak with an Expert: See a fitness expert if you're new to exercising or if you have any medical issues.

These exercises and advice will help you develop a strong, steady core that will help you in all of your physical activities. Keep in mind that core strength is about building a strong foundation for your body's safe and efficient movement, not merely about having a toned abdomen.

CHAPTER 8: Including Somatic Activities in Everyday Life

Somatic activities are a great way to improve your mind-body connection on a regular basis. To relieve stress, start with easy techniques like gradual muscle relaxation and attentive breathing. Incorporate tai chi or mild yoga to increase your strength and flexibility. Grounding and body awareness activities on a daily basis may improve physical and emotional well-being, resulting in a more balanced and thoughtful way of living.

Workplace Somatics

A useful strategy for bringing movement and body awareness into the workplace is somatics. This may result in better posture, lower stress levels, and higher output. This is a thorough handbook on incorporating somatic techniques into your daily workday:

Knowing the Somatics
The emphasis of somatics, a branch of bodywork and wellbeing, is on inward bodily sensation and perception. It's about learning to move with awareness and purpose and getting back in touch with your body's feelings.

Advantages of Somatic Practices in the Workplace

Decreases Physical Strain: Working in an office often causes stress and strain. Somatic exercises are particularly effective in relieving pain in the neck, shoulders, and back.
Improves Mental Clarity: Somatic activities may improve mental clarity by easing physical tension, which improves attention and judgment.
Promotes Emotional Well-Being: Mindful movement may aid in stress reduction and the development of serenity.

Office-Friendly Somatic Exercises:

1. Sitting Pelvic Shifts: To activate your core and reduce lower back strain, gently move your pelvis forth and backward while sitting.
2. Shoulder Rolls: To relieve tension in your shoulders, raise them up near your ears, roll them back, and then lower.
3. Neck Stretches: To relieve stiffness in your neck, tilt your head from side to side and hold each pose for a few breaths.
4. Hand and Wrist Stretches: To stretch your hands and ease wrist tension from typing, extend your arms and slowly draw back on your fingers.

Integrating Somatics into Your Da

- Morning Routine: Before starting work, do a body scan and take note of any tense spots.

- Micro-Breaks: During the day, take brief pauses to engage in somatic activities, such as ideokinesis to release weight or tactile activation to reenergize.
- Lunchtime Movement: Make use of a portion of your lunch break to engage in a more extensive somatic exercise, such a light yoga pose or a complete body stretch.
- End-of-Day Wind Down: To help you transition from work to home life, end your workday with a relaxing somatic activity, such as aware breathing or a sitting pelvic shift.

Building an Ergonomic Workspace

- Comfortable Posture: Make sure your chair and workstation allow you to sit comfortably with your feet flat on the floor and your screen at eye level.
- Reminders: Make sure to schedule frequent somatic breaks by setting reminders on your phone or computer.
- Community: Whether in person or digitally, invite coworkers to participate in group somatic sessions.

Safety and Considerations

1. Personal Comfort: Make sure you're always moving in a pain-free and comfortable range.
2. Expert Counseling: To guarantee correct technique, if you're new to somatics, think about getting advice from a specialist.

67 Somatic Exercises For Weight Loss

Somatic exercises might help you establish a more body-friendly and attentive work atmosphere in your business. This enhances your physical well-being and makes your workplace more pleasurable and productive.

Travelers' Somatics

Numerous techniques that concentrate on the interior feelings and sensations of the body are part of somatics. These techniques may be very helpful for travelers in controlling the physical aches and strains brought on by travel.

Benefits of Somatic Practices for Travelers
- Improves Physical Comfort: Somatic exercises may help release tension and enhance circulation. Extended sitting times can make people stiff.
- Improves Travel Experience: You may travel more sensibly and thoroughly by being in the present moment when you are more in touch with your body.

Travelers' Somatic Exercises
1. Seated Stretches: To maintain the body fluid throughout lengthy flights or rides, gently twist your neck, shrug your shoulders, and stretch your wrists.
2. Breathing Techniques: To lower stress and soothe the nervous system, practice deep belly breathing.
3. Mindful Walking: When venturing into unfamiliar territory, pay attention to the feelings and motions of your body.

4. Grounding Exercises: After a long day of traveling, try feeling the stability of the earth under your feet. This may be a relaxing exercise.

Integrating Somatics into Travel Routines

- Pre-Travel: Before embarking on your travel, do a body scan to find any tense regions.
- In-Transit: To keep your body alert and avoid stiffness, do somatic exercises while sitting or during layovers.
- Post-Travel: After arriving at your location, restore your body and mind with a more thorough somatic regimen.

Building a Travel-Friendly Somatic Kit

- Portable Tools: Bring tools to help with your somatic activities, such as a massage ball, resistance bands, or a travel yoga mat.
- Digital Resources: Get applications or audio instructions that provide mobile somatic exercises.
- Comfort Items: To improve your physical comfort while traveling, pack a neck cushion or lumbar support.

Safety and Considerations

- Space Constraints: Adjust workouts to the available space while being aware of your surroundings.
- Cultural Sensitivity: Show consideration for regional traditions and customs while doing somatic exercises in public areas.

- Expert Advice: Before your travel, speak with a somatic practitioner if you have any particular health concerns.

You may preserve physical well-being and improve your travel experience by including somatic workouts in your regimen. Traveling for pleasure or business may both benefit from somatic practices, which can help you arrive at your location feeling rejuvenated and eager to explore.

Establishing a Customized Somatic Practice

Developing a customized somatic regimen entails adjusting body-awareness exercises to your unique requirements and way of living. Using a holistic approach may result in better physical health, less stress, and a stronger sense of self-awareness. To develop a somatic practice that appeals to you, follow these steps:
 A customized somatic regimen is a series of movements intended to assist you in becoming aware of the particular rhythms and requirements of your body. It's about identifying exercises that improve mobility, relieve stress, and foster awareness.

Personalized Somatic Routine Benefits
- Designed to Meet Specific Needs- targets certain body parts that are tense or unbalanced.
- Adaptable and Flexible: may be changed to accommodate any timetable, whether you have five minutes or eight hours.

- Encourages Self-Awareness: promotes a greater comprehension of the messages sent by your body and how to react to them.

How to Establish Your Somatic Rhythm

1. Assess Your Body: To begin, check your body for tight, uncomfortable, or imbalanced regions.

2. Set Specific Objectives: Identify the results you want to get from your program, such as better pain management, less stress, or enhanced flexibility.

3. Select Your Workouts: Choose somatic workouts that are beneficial to your body and help you achieve your objectives. Think of exercises from Feldenkrais, yoga, or tai chi.

4. Make a Schedule: Choose the days and times that you'll practice your program. In order to reap the rewards, consistency is essential.

5. Monitor Progress: As you interact with your routine, record changes in your body and mind in a notebook.

Model Personalized Somatic Routine

- Awakening: Stretching gently and breathing mindfully to arouse the body.
- Midday: Somatic desk exercises to release tension from work.
- Evening: A soothing series of exercises to get you ready for a good night's sleep.

- Including Mindfulness--Mindful Breathing: During activities, use your breath as an anchor to help you stay mindful of the here and now.
- Visualization: To improve the somatic experience, see tension dissipating with each movement.
- Body Sensing: Develop a close relationship with yourself by being aware of the feelings in your body when you move.

Customizing Your Schedule

- Pay Attention to Your Body: Modify your daily schedule in accordance with how your body feels. On some days, you may want to do more active exercises, while on other days, you might need to do more mild ones.
- Ask for Professional Advice: Refine your practice and make sure you're practicing safely and successfully by working with a somatic practitioner.

Safety and Concerns

- Avoid Pain: Pain should never be experienced when doing somatic exercises. Change the exercise or omit it if you are uncomfortable.
- Progress Gradually: As your body adjusts, begin with basic exercises and work your way up to more difficult ones.

You may enjoy a practice that improves your mental and emotional well-being in addition to improving your physical well-being by designing a customized somatic regimen. A more peaceful and balanced existence may result from this path of self-discovery and nurturing.

CHAPTER 9: Diet and Physiology

Somatics and nutrition work together to improve overall wellness. The body needs proper nourishment to sustain somatic activities, which increase movement efficiency and physical awareness. In line with somatic principles, mindful eating promotes awareness of hunger and fullness signals and results in a diet that is well-balanced. When combined, they create a synergistic interaction that enhances mental clarity and physical vitality both necessary for a healthy mind-body connection.

Eating Conscientiously

Being totally present and involved when eating, concentrating on the sensory aspects and feelings connected to food, is the practice of mindful eating. This is a thorough handbook on developing mindful eating practices:

The foundation of mindful eating is mindfulness, a kind of meditation that entails giving the current moment your whole attention. When it comes to eating, it refers to appreciating every taste and understanding the impact that food has on your body and emotions.

- Improves Sensory Appreciation: Meals may be made more pleasurable by focusing on the flavor, texture, and scent of the food.
- Promotes Digestive Health: Slow, mindful eating helps enhance nutritional absorption and digestion.
- Controls Appetite: Being aware of your hunger and fullness signals might help you avoid overindulging in food.
- Reduces Stress: Eating mindfully may be a relaxing habit that eases tension and anxiety related to food.

Conscious Eating Principles

1. Activate Every Sense: Take note of the tastes, textures, noises, colors, and scents of your meal.
2. Chew Thoroughly: Give your meal a good chewing experience to fully experience the tastes and facilitate digestion.
3. Remove Distractions: Switch off the television and store your electronics so that you can concentrate only on eating.
4. Honor Your Hunger: Don't eat out of boredom, stress, or habit; instead, eat when you are physically hungry.
5. Appreciate Your Food: Give thanks for the journey your food has gone from farm to plate.

Mindful Eating Practices

- Mindful Check-In: Evaluate your hunger and mood in advance of eating.

75 Somatic Exercises For Weight Loss

- Portion Control: Reduce the quantity you serve yourself to prevent mindless overindulgence.
- Mindful Pauses: Throughout your meal, take brief breaks from using your cutlery to consider how satiated you are.
- Conscious Decisions: Choose foods that will feed and fulfill your body.

Building a Mindful Eating Environment

- Sweetheart Scene: Establish a serene and cozy dining space that promotes pleasure and rest.
- -Regular Meal Times: To help control your body's hunger signals, establish a regular mealtime schedule.
- -Social Engagement: You may improve the dining experience by conversing with others while sharing food.

Overcoming Difficulties

Handling desires: Choose how you want to react to desires and acknowledge them without passing judgment.
-Emotional Eating: Investigate your feelings via mindfulness in order to identify healthy coping mechanisms.

- Resources for Mindful Eating--Books and Guides: Seek for reading material that provides more in-depth explanations of mindful eating techniques.
- Classes and programs: Take part in programs that provide practical experience in mindful eating.

- Apps and Online Tools: Make use of electronic tools that provide guided mindful eating activities.

You may change your connection with food from one of mindless intake to one of deliberate delight by adopting mindful eating. It's a path that enhances your mental and emotional health in addition to your physical health.

Foods that Encourage Physical Activity

Foods that increase vitality, lower inflammation, and strengthen the body's innate capacity for self-regulation are supportive of somatic practice. This is a thorough tutorial on body nutrition to support your somatic exercises:

Foods that meet the body's demands, enhance mental-body integration, and foster overall wellbeing are the main emphasis of somatic-friendly diet, which is crucial to somatic activities.

Energy-Boosting Foods
Key Nutritional Components for Somatic Practice: To maintain energy levels throughout your somatic workouts, including complex carbohydrates and proteins.-Anti-Inflammatory Foods: Choose foods high in omega-3 fatty acids, antioxidants, and phytonutrients to help decrease inflammation and assist in recovery2.-Gut-Health Foods: For general health, maintain a healthy gut microbiota by eating foods rich in fiber, such as fruits, vegetables, and whole grains.

77 Somatic Exercises For Weight Loss

Included Foods
1. Leafy Greens: Packed with vitamins and minerals, spinach, kale, and other greens aid in muscle growth and recuperation.
2. Nuts and Seeds: Flaxseeds, chia seeds, and almonds are good sources of protein and healthy fats for long-term energy.
3. Whole Grains: Complex carbohydrates are provided by quinoa, brown rice, and oats, which provide sustained energy.
4. Lean Proteins: Fish, tofu, chicken, and beans aid in the development and repair of muscular tissue.
5. Fruits: Rich in fiber and antioxidants, berries, oranges, and apples may help fight oxidative stress.

Hydration and Somatic Practice
1. Water: Maintaining joint lubrication and muscle flexibility requires drinking enough water, which is crucial for somatic movement.
2. Herbal Teas: Some teas, such as those infused with ginger or turmeric, have relaxing and anti-inflammatory properties.

Somatics and Mindful Eating
1. Listen to Your Body: Observe how various meals impact your mood and level of energy. To complement your somatic practice, modify your food appropriately.
2. Lunch Timing: To ensure you have adequate energy without feeling burdened down, think about having a small, healthy lunch or snack before your practice.

3. Developing a Somatic Nutrition Plan--Personalization: Adjust your nutrition plan to suit your specific requirements, accounting for any dietary preferences or limitations.

4. Balance: To support all facets of your health, strive for a balanced diet that contains a range of nutrients.

5. Consultation: If necessary, seek the advice of a nutritionist who can assist you in formulating a plan that enhances your somatic regimen.

You may increase the advantages of your workouts and foster a stronger connection between your body and mind by putting an emphasis on foods that assist somatic practice.

Exercise requires proper hydration since it affects both performance and recuperation. This is a thorough tutorial explaining the importance of staying hydrated and how to do so while exercising:

The Significance of Hydration in Exercise

1. Controls Body Temperature: By encouraging sweat production, which lowers body temperature during vigorous exercise, adequate hydration helps control body temperature.

2. Lubricates Joints: Consuming enough fluids keeps joints lubricated and lowers the chance of damage.

3. Transports Nutrients: Water is necessary to provide energy, carry nutrients to cells, and aid in healing.

Knowing Your Electrolytes

1. Balance Fluids: Electrolytes such as magnesium, potassium, and sodium assist in maintaining the proper balance of fluids throughout the body.

2. Support muscular Function: They are essential for cramp prevention and muscular contractions.

3. Aid in Recovery: Restoring electrolytes after physical activity promotes a speedy recuperation and lessens fatigue.

Exercise Hydration Strategies

1. Pre exercise: Sip 17–20 ounces of water two to three hours before to beginning your exercise.

2. While Exercising: Drink 7–10 ounces of water every 10–20 minutes to replenish fluids lost via perspiration.

3. Post-Workout: Replace lost fluids with 16–24 ounces of water for each pound of exercise.

Dehydration Signs

1. Dark Urine: Clearly indicating that you need to increase your fluid intake.

2. Dehydrated and Parched Mouth: Your body's signals to drink more water.

3. Weakness and Lightheadedness: May arise from the body not getting enough water.

Selecting Hydration Fluids

1. Water: The optimal option for the majority of workouts, particularly those that last less than 60 minutes.

2. Sports Drinks: Because they are heavy in carbs and electrolytes, they are helpful for endurance exercises or intense workouts that last longer than an hour.

3. Coconut Water: A healthier substitute for sports drinks that provides electrolytes without as much added sugar.

Hydration Tips

1. Monitor Fluid Loss: To determine how much fluid you've lost during activity, weigh yourself both before and after.

2. Pay Attention to Your Body: Since thirst is a late sign of dehydration, it's important to consistently consume fluids rather than waiting to feel thirsty.

3. Avoid Overhydration: Hyponatremia, a condition when the blood's salt levels fall too low, may result from consuming excessive amounts of water.

Diet and Hydration

1. Balanced Meals: To help with hydration, include fruits and vegetables in your diet that are rich in water content.

2. Limit Diuretics: Drinks such as alcohol and coffee should be limited since they might cause fluid loss.

Personal Hydration Plan

1. Individual Needs: Depending on your age, weight, degree of fitness, and the environment, you may require different amounts of water.

2. Expert Counsel: Speak with a dietician or other medical expert to develop a customized hydration strategy that fits your lifestyle and workout routine.

Understanding the importance of hydration during exercise and putting these tips into practice can help you make sure your body is ready for action, which will improve performance and hasten the healing process.

CHAPTER 10: Monitoring Your Development

A crucial first step toward success and personal development is setting reasonable objectives. Here is a thorough how-to guide for creating ambitious but attainable goals:

Knowing What Realistic Goals Are
A realistic aim is one that is difficult yet doable in a certain amount of time and with the resources at hand. They encourage you to develop while positioning you for success by striking a balance between desire and pragmatism.

SMART Framework Overview
The SMART criteria are among the best tools for creating realistic objectives.
-Specific: Clearly state your objectives.
-Measurable: Choose a method for monitoring your development.
-Achievable: Verify that you can accomplish the objective.
-Relevant: Make sure the aim is in line with your long-term goals and values.
-Time-bound: Establish a completion date[12].

How to Set Reasonable Objectives

1. Self-Assessment: To help you define goals, consider your prior experiences, limitations, and strengths.

2. Research: Compile data to determine what is needed to accomplish your objective.

3. -Resource Evaluation: Take into account the resources you now possess as well as those you may need.

4. Action Plan: Establish a defined schedule and divide your objective into smaller, more doable activities.

5. Adaptability: Be ready to modify your objectives as conditions change.·.

Achieve Your Goals

1. Write Them Down: Writing down your objectives strengthens your dedication and gives them a concrete form.

2. Visualize Success: Envision the result and the actions required to get there.

3. Track Progress: Evaluate your progress toward your objectives on a regular basis.

4. Remain Driven: Convince yourself of the significance of the objective.

5. Seek Support: Never be afraid to approach peers or mentors for advice or assistance.

Common Pitfalls to Avoid

- Overambitious Goals: Aiming too high could result in fatigue and dissatisfaction.

- Vague Objectives: It is challenging to take decisive action in the absence of clarity.
- Neglecting Personal Limits: Setting unachievable objectives is a consequence of ignoring your own limitations.
- Lack of Patience: Expecting quick fixes might leave you disappointed since real transformation takes time.

Preserving Equilibrium

Setting objectives that take into account your physical and emotional well-being is just as vital as pushing yourself. Make sure your objectives support a healthy lifestyle and don't jeopardize your happiness or health.

By adhering to these recommendations and using the SMART framework, you may create attainable objectives that inspire you to proceed and acknowledge the significant achievements along the route. Always keep in mind that the process of reaching a goal is just as significant as the final destination.

Maintaining a Journal of Somatic Exercise

A thoughtful practice that may improve your entire somatic experience and help you better understand how your body reacts to movement is keeping a somatic exercise diary. This is a thorough advice on keeping an excellent somatic exercise journal:

Knowing Why You Should Keep a Somatic Exercise Journal
You may keep a somatic exercise diary to document your thoughts, feelings, and bodily experiences before to, during, and after somatic exercises. It assists you in monitoring your development, identifying trends, and drawing parallels between your somatic practice and everyday life.

Advantages of Maintaining a Somatic Exercise Journal
- Improved Body Awareness: Putting your experiences in writing will help you become more conscious of your physical motions and feelings.
- Emotional Clarity: You may recognize and go with feelings associated with your somatic practice by keeping a journal.
- Personal Development: Reading back over your journal entries may help you see patterns, inclinations, and areas in which you still need to improve.

Introduction to Somatic Exercise Record-Keeping
1. Select a Medium: Make the decision on whether you would rather keep your journal in a conventional notebook, a digital file, or a specific app.
2. Create a Routine: Choose a regular journaling time, such just after your somatic exercises.
3. Create a Comfortable Space: Locate a peaceful, cozy area where you may write and ponder.

What to Write in Your Journal

- Time and Date: Note the time of the somatic session.
- Physical feelings: Take note of any unique bodily releases, tensions, or feelings.
- Emotional Responses: Explain the feelings you had during the exercise.
- Thoughts and Reflections: Jot down any ideas or realizations that came to mind.
- Exercises Completed: Enumerate the precise somatic exercises you completed.
- Practice Duration: Note the length of each somatic session.
- Environmental Factors: Address any outside influences, including noise or interruptions, that may have affected your practice.

Journaling Techniques

- Body Scanning: Take a brief physical inventory before writing to become aware of any feelings or sensations.
- Free Writing: Don't bother about grammar or structure; just write whatever comes to mind.
- Prompted Entries: Examine certain aspects of your somatic experience by using diary prompts.

Reviewing and Thinking Back on Your Journal

1. Regular Reviews: Schedule time once a week or once a month to go over your journal entries and consider how far you've come.

2. Identify Patterns: Examine your somatic practice for any reoccurring themes or shifts.

3. Modify Your Practice: Make improvements to your somatic exercises based on the observations you make in your diary.

Personalization and Privacy

1. Keep It Secret: Your somatic exercise log is a private piece of writing. If you'd rather keep your reflections to yourself, make sure it's stored in a secret location.

2. Customize Your diary: Add drawings, sayings, or anything else that inspires you to make your diary really yours.

Difficulties and Solution

1. Regularity: If you struggle to journal on a regular basis, consider setting reminders or combining journaling with another everyday routine.

2. Depth of Reflection: If you find it difficult to move beyond cursory observations, think about attending somatic journaling seminars or participating in guided journaling.

Keeping a somatic exercise diary allows you to establish a vital tool for understanding the mind-body connection and for personal growth. It's a technique that enhances your somatic workouts and helps you live a more contemplative and thoughtful life.

Determining Success Apart from Scale

There is much more to measuring fitness and health performance than just looking at points on a scale. It's about realizing the many ways that adopting a healthy lifestyle enhances your body and mind. Here's a thorough how-to manual for measuring achievement above and beyond the scale:

Knowing Success Above and Beyond the Scale

Fitness and health success have several facets. Even while weight may be measured, it's not the only or even the most significant measure of development. Elements such as bone density, muscular mass, and general health are important.

Alternative Metrics of Achievement

- Body Composition: Gaining muscle while reducing fat may not show up on the scale, but it will greatly enhance your body and metabolism2.
- Fitness Levels: Progress is plainly shown by gains in strength, endurance, and flexibility.
- Energy and Stamina: Better health is indicated by increased energy and stamina for everyday tasks or exercise.
- Mental Well-Being: A positive outlook, improved stress reduction techniques, and a feeling of accomplishment all play a part in total success.
- Health Markers: Notable improvements in blood pressure, cholesterol, and blood sugar regulation have been achieved2.

89 Somatic Exercises For Weight Loss

- Non-Scale Victories (NSVs)--Clothing Fit: A measurable indicator of improvement is whether or if clothes fit better or a size down.
- Physical Measurements: Measurements of your arms, legs, waist, and hips might reveal improvement that is not shown by your scale.
- Quality of Sleep: Recuperation and overall health depend heavily on getting better sleep.
- Improved Habits: Choosing better foods and exercising regularly are accomplishments in and of themselves.

Creating Practical Objectives

SMART Objectives: Establish Targets that go Beyond Just Losing Weight and go Specific, Measurable, Achievable, Relevant, and Time-bound..-Personal Milestones: Honor accomplishments in workouts, longer strolls, or any previously difficult activity.

- Tracking Progress--Journaling: Record your physical and emotional well-being in a diary as you progress toward fitness.
- Photographs: To visually record your trip and compare changes over time, take frequent images.
- Fitness applications: Track your steps, exercises, and other fitness-related data using applications.

Holistic Health Indicators

- Nutrition: Observing how certain meals effect your body's reaction and how it impacts your energy levels.
- Hydration: Observing changes in drinking habits, which have an impact on digestion, skin health, and other areas.
- Social and Emotional: Acknowledging improved emotional reactions and social interactions as a component of a healthy way of living.

Difficulties and Overcoming Them

- Plateaus: Recognize that you will inevitably reach a weight reduction plateau and concentrate on other areas of improvement.
- Mindset Shift: Develop an appreciation for progress in all its manifestations, not simply in terms of weight reduction.

Success has several facets and is individualized. Through a variety of progress measurements, you may get a more realistic and motivating image of your health journey. Always keep in mind that each good change, no matter how little, is a step in the direction of a happier and healthier you[12].

CHAPTER 11: Overcoming Obstacles

It may be difficult to overcome plateaus in any area of life—weight loss, fitness, work, or personal development. When efforts are put out and development seems to stop, a plateau occurs. This is a thorough tutorial on overcoming and navigating through plateaus:

Comprehending Stagnations
A plateau occurs when there is no discernible advancement for an extended length of time. It's the sense of being trapped in one's profession without moving forward; in fitness, it's the stalling of strength or endurance gains; in weight reduction, it's the inability to move the scale.

The body or mind becomes used to a routine, and the initial pace of improvement is not long-term sustainable. This is one of the -
Common Causes of Plateaus
1. Complacency: Getting too comfortable and not pushing oneself to the limit.
2. Inefficient Strategies: Keeping up with tactics that aren't working anymore.

Methods for Breaking Through Plateaus

1. Reevaluate and Modify Objectives: Verify that your objectives remain SMART (Specific, Measurable, Achievable, Relevant, Time-bound).

2. Change Your Approach: Vary up your regimen by trying out different workouts, making dietary changes, or taking on new responsibilities at work.

3. Monitor Progress: Maintain an extensive record of your actions and results to pinpoint areas that want improvement.

4. Intensity: Occasionally, exerting more effort or making activities more challenging may spur progress.

5. Rest and Recover: Occasionally, taking a break is essential to rejuvenate and return stronger[1]

Mindset and Plateaus

1. Stay Positive: Remind yourself that obstacles are a natural part of the trip and have an optimistic attitude.

2. Be Patient: Recognize that patience is essential and that development is not always linear.

3. Learn and Grow: Take advantage of the plateau to refine your skills and get fresh perspectives about yourself.

Looking for Assistance

1. Expert Counseling: Speak with professionals who can provide tailored guidance, such as career coaches, personal trainers, or nutritionists.

2. Community Support: Talk to others who are traveling similar paths in order to get advice and inspiration.

Measuring Success Differently

1. Non-Scale Victories: Seek for other indications of development, such more vitality, better-fitting clothing, or improved abilities.

2. Holistic Health: Take into account gains in psychological and emotional stability as success markers.

Maintaining Momentum

1. Appreciate Small Wins: To maintain a positive attitude, recognize and appreciate even the tiniest accomplishments.

2. Modify Your Expectations: Establish attainable goals and be honest about the pace of development.

A plateau is a normal component of any process of development. You may overcome them and keep moving forward on your road to success by comprehending their causes and putting useful ideas into practice. Recall that every plateau presents a chance for self-evaluation, education, and strength-building.

Physical Components of Emotional Eating

Maintaining Motivation

It may be difficult to maintain motivation, particularly when confronted with setbacks or when the thrill of starting anything new wanes. But maintaining development and reaching objectives need motivation. This is a thorough manual on maintaining motivation that includes useful advice on maintaining momentum:

Comprehending Drive

The energy that starts, directs, and sustains goal-oriented activities is known as motivation. It's what drives you to act and persevere in the face of difficulties. Two primary categories of motivation exist:

1. Intrinsic Motivation: Motivated by self-satisfaction and internal benefits.

2. Extrinsic Motivation: Motivated by benefits from outside sources or by a desire to stay out of trouble.

Action Items for Remaining Motivated

1. Create a Plan: Divide your objectives into smaller, more manageable tasks and assign due dates for each.

2. Set Clear Goals: Specify what you want to accomplish using specific, measurable, achievable, relevant, and time-bound (SMART) criteria.

3. Track Your Progress: Keep a log of your accomplishments, no matter how small, to stay motivated.

4. Find Your Why: To stay connected to your motives, comprehend the underlying causes of your ambitions.

5. Create a Support Network: Be in the company of individuals who uplift and support you in your endeavors.

6. Celebrate Small Wins: Give yourself a pat on the back for the accomplishments you make along the way.

7. Stay Flexible: Be open to modifying your plans and strategies as necessary to stay on course.

8. Maintain a Positive Attitude: Foster optimism and resilience to overcome setbacks.

9. Visualize Success: Visualize reaching your goals and the feelings that come with it to motivate action.

10. Stay Healthy: Take care of your physical well-being with a healthy diet, exercise, and rest to maintain energy levels.

11. Learn from Setbacks: Utilize setbacks as teaching opportunities and feedback to improve your tactics.

12. Limitate Distractions: Establish a workspace that encourages productivity and focus.

13. Practice Gratitude: Ponder the things you're thankful for in your life.

14. Seek Inspiration: Watch films, read books, or tune in to podcasts that inspire you to keep moving ahead.

15. Take on New Challenges: Venture outside your comfort zone to maintain interest and engagement.

Removing Typical Barriers

1. Delaying: Address it by dividing work into manageable chunks and beginning with the simplest portion2.

2. Lack of Energy: Make sure you're getting enough rest, moving about, and eating a healthy diet to help with this.

3. Self-Doubt: Overcome this by restating your skills and accomplishments from the past2.

Maintaining motivation is an ever-changing process that calls for constant work and adjustment. You may retain motivation over time by putting these suggestions into practice and being dedicated to your objectives. Recall that individual motivation varies, thus what motivates one person could not motivate another. Choose what speaks to you and incorporate it into your path to success.

CONCLUSION

As we come to an end on this life-changing adventure, my goal is that the book's pages have functioned as a compass, pointing you in the direction of your goals. The real value of this book is not only what you read, but how you apply its ideas to your everyday life. It is a vessel loaded with success tactics, life lessons learned, and inspiration to strive for greatness.

The path to reaching your ideal goal requires persistent work and unshakable dedication. Allow this book to be your reliable friend, a wellspring of motivation when things appear difficult and a guiding light when uncertainty obscures your judgment. Although the information on these pages is a strong tool, action is the only way to fully realize its potential.

As the reader, I implore you to keep this book from collecting dust on a shelf. Rather, let it to collect the traces of repeated use. Go over its chapters again, consider its teachings, and put its suggestions into practice. Establish quantifiable objectives and track your progress. No matter how little your wins may be, acknowledge them and take lessons from your failures. They are not mistakes; rather, they are milestones on route to achievement.

Recall that achieving your ideal goal is a personal challenge that is exclusive to you. Though you are the explorer, this book serves as a map. Have faith in your skills, capitalize on your advantages, and work on your shortcomings. Remain driven, maintain your curiosity, and most importantly, remain loyal to your goal.

I'll close by expressing my deepest hopes for your achievement. I hope the knowledge you have acquired acts as a basis for you to create a successful and happy life. Take this book, put it to good use, and go on with self-assurance toward your goals. Your ideal target is right in front of you.